Simple Guide to CBD
Not All Hemp Products Are Created Equal!

Maggie Hall

Disclaimer: No information contained in this booklet is intended to make any claims about CBD or claims about any products mentioned, and no inference of such should be taken. Reviews cited in the booklet are the opinions of the user, and reflect their personal experience with the products mentioned. Research cited or mentioned is the opinion of the researchers and should not be taken as a claim for any products mentioned in this booklet.

DEDICATION

I dedicate this to my many inspirational mentors
throughout this life,
and to ALL creatures, great and small. . .

My numerous human mentors and animal teachers have
been wise, and very patient with me. I thank you for
nurturing me along. Now it is time to give back
to you a million-fold!

CONTENTS

Introduction   Page 3

1   What is the Difference Between   Page 4
Marijuana and Hemp?

2   MAPS/NORML Vaporizer Study   Page 6

3   Health Benefits of CBD   Page 8

4   The Financial Side of Cannabis   Page 17

5   What You Should Know About   Page 20
Your CBD Products

6   You Need To Know!   Page 29

7   Care and Devotion for the Plants   Page 32
and the People

8   Why Does It Matter Which Carrier   Page 38
You Mix It With?

9   What is the Why?   Page 42

ACKNOWLEDGMENT

I would love to thank all of my dogs, horses, cats, and the parrots and wildlife who have come into my life to be teachers and guides. You are amazing!

And I give gratitude to my family, who are my shining example of unconditional love.

My abundant thanks and appreciation to Imbue Botanicals' Dan Iannotte and the entire Team at Imbue. Through all the trials and the many years, they have persevered and succeeded.

The highest quality premium CBD from organic hemp grown in Colorado is now available to all of us, and we are very grateful to Imbue Botanicals, for taking the extra time and expense and raising the bar for all CBD companies in the future.

Someday we will all look back and say how thankful we are that we could be a part of this movement, making it possible for millions of mammals'
healing and restoration to perfect health.

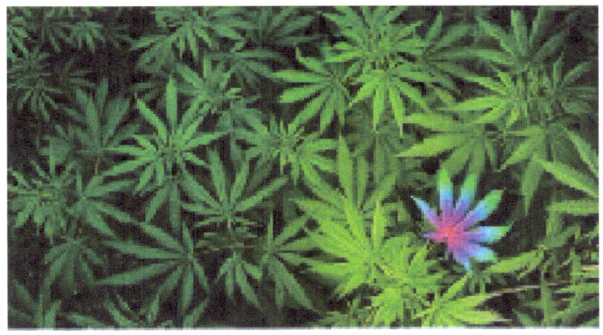

Simple Guide to CBD - Not All Hemp Products Are Created Equal!

Introduction

I believe that people have the right to know the truth behind the production and processing of products that they and their animals are ingesting. CBD (cannabidiol) is a healing compound in the cannabis plant; just one of over a hundred active compounds called cannabinoids. It is not psychoactive - and it has wide acclaim due to its therapeutic properties.

People don't need to get a medical marijuana card and they can still benefit from the healing power of the cannabis plant by using CBD products in many forms (tinctures, capsules, lotions and salves, to name a few). We will mainly focus on CBD in this book. Many people are hard at work, searching for a quality company to purchase CBD products from. They are out there!

CHAPTER ONE

What is the Difference Between Marijuana and Hemp?

Both marijuana and hemp are of the same plant species, Cannabis sativa L. They are considered to be "Cannabis Cousins".

Hemp is typically bred for industrial and food uses such as oils, seeds, supplements, topical ointments, fiber for clothing, construction, and much more. The whole hemp plant can be used, not just the flowers. It has either zero or trace amounts of THC, the psychoactive cannabinoid. Hemp is a wonderful assimilable source of plant protein.

Marijuana has been bred for high amounts of THC and usually lower amounts of CBD. It is short and bushy to encourage more flowers, which are the desirable part of the plant. Hemp plants are very tall and sturdy, and have less branching than the smaller marijuana plants.

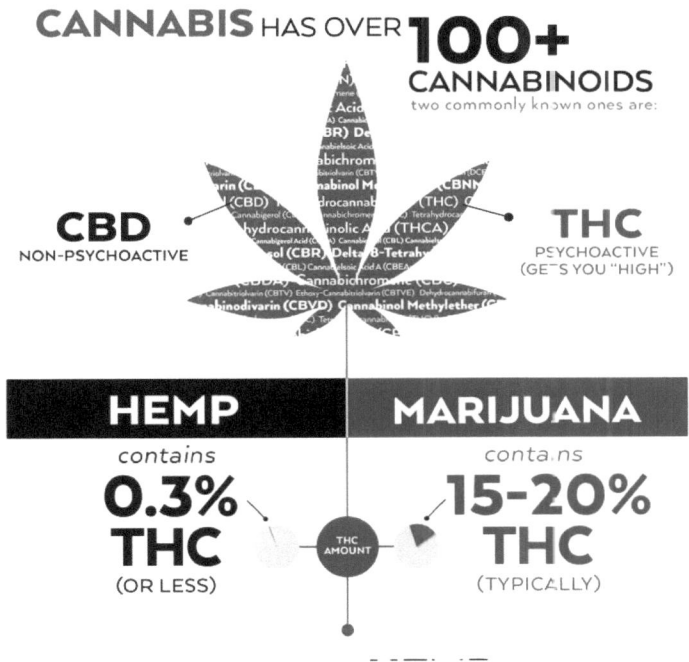

Diagram courtesy of Charlotte's Web

CHAPTER TWO

MAPS/NORML Vaporizer Study

While working for MAPS (Multi-disciplinary Association for Psychedelic Studies) as an editor, we were publishing the results of the MAPS/NORML study. The research proved that vaporizers reduce the toxins in marijuana smoke. "MAPS and NORML sponsored the study in the hopes of helping medical marijuana patients and others (to) reduce the health risks of smoking marijuana..... Output from the vaporizer was analyzed and compared to smoke produced by burning the sample..... Carbon monoxide and smoke tars were both qualitatively reduced by the vaporizer..."
Dale Gieringer, PhD.; NORML California State Coordinator;
http://www.maps.org/news-letters/v11n1/pdf/11120gie.pdf

I am a strong advocate for the use of medical marijuana. I have become a devoted supporter of CBD products as well, especially for children, the elderly, and anyone who is seeking the health benefits of cannabis without the altered states associated with ingesting THC

(Tetrahydrocannabinol, the psychoactive compound in cannabis). Also, some patients need much more CBD and much less THC, depending on what it is they are treating.

In the US, marijuana is still a Schedule 1 drug, putting it in the same category as heroin. This is archaic and it is up to the public to demand that they have the right to grow cannabis themselves if they want to, and to use it either recreationally or as a medicine. Luckily, CBD has broader legal footing and many companies will ship to all 50 states.

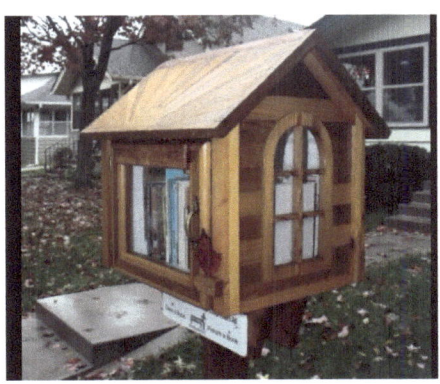

CHAPTER THREE

Health Benefits of CBD

It is easy to find studies online about the research going on with CBD and a quick google search will keep you busy for hours. Do your own research and try the capsules or tinctures yourself to see what results you get. We all have our own "chemistry lab" in our bodies, and we all react differently to different things. That's why we have to try out what dose works the best for us individually.

There are wide applications for the use of CBD. As time goes on and people get experience with how it affects them personally, more and more anecdotal stories accumulate. Personally, I have had three years of acute hip pain disappear and along with that, have had a bad knee injury completely heal.

It also gives me a very positive feeling, and I know it is giving me a balance in my body that I believe will be working prophylactically to prevent any physical issues in the future. I am so happy to hear other peoples' stories, and they consistently report that the Imbue CBD is helping with a wide variety of ailments.

"I had my dad on your Health-25 (25mg capsules) prior to and during chemotherapy for recurrent bladder cancer. The doctors said there was about a 25% chance that chemo would be effective in Dad's case, so we thought adding CBD might improve the odds. I'm thrilled to report that Dad was at the oncologist earlier in the week and the doctor could find no visible evidence of the cancer! I'm going to keep Dad on the Health-10 (10mg capsules) going forward as a prophylactic measure. Thank you!"

Shelley P. ~ October 9, 2016

Wow! Where do I even start?? Imbue has been a GAME CHANGER for me!! I started taking the 25mg capsules about three months ago. A couple of months prior to that, I came off prescription medication I had been taking for anxiety. Although I was able to get off the medication by myself... I wish I had begun taking CBD sooner!!

As soon as I started taking the 25mg CBD capsules, I felt so much more confident, energized and capable! I was able to go out with friends without experiencing intense anxiety or stress. I felt more confident in my work and I started speaking up for myself more.

As someone who has dealt with depression off and on for 10+ years, has tried several anti-depressants and anxiety medications... I have never experienced results as life-changing as the ones I have experienced from Imbue. Although I do have some hard days here and there, they are nothing close to the extreme depressive episodes I experienced before. Imbue's 25mg capsules really help to elevate my mood and keep me in a more positive state.

Thank you for creating this wonderful product!!

Ashley Carvahlo – June 21, 2017 - Regarding the Health 25, 25mg capsules

"Amazing stuff - I fostered Hurley, a lab mix, in 2011 and soon realized why his previous owner got tired of him. This dog is very loving but has issues - fence jumping, anxiety over sprinklers, lightning, fireworks, and separation. Fast forward to 2017 and I hear about CBD oil, and decided to give it a try.

After a couple of days, Hurley is a different dog - he's calm and doesn't jump the fence! He will calmly sit when I leave, and ignores loud noises. We had some severe thunderstorms last night with nearby lightning strikes, and Hurley just sat on the couch with me and then rolled over for a belly rub. He used to be cowering and trying to dig an escape tunnel. If your dog has anxieties like Hurley, you need to try this."

Steve – May 21, 2017 - Regarding K9 Comfort tincture for dogs

"Back in late October, my 14 y/o male pit mix got very sick. One day, he had been a little lethargic on our hike but was otherwise completely normal. The next morning, he woke up, ate breakfast and promptly projectile vomited it back up. This went on for 3 days. I put him on super mild food, to no avail. He didn't want to walk and he had dropped about 10 pounds.

I took him to my vet on the 3rd night and the vet ran a number of tests which established that he had pancreatitis and that there was a hole in a tumor in his chest that was leaking fluid into his chest cavity. She said that it was very unlikely that he would be with us through the weekend and that we should start making arrangements.

I called Dan Iannotte, who happens to be a close friend, just to let him know what was going on - and he sent me a bottle of CBD oil and told me to give him a capsule daily and that it would help with his pain at the very least. So I did.

It is now the end of February and Astro is better than ever! He takes CBD once a day with breakfast and gets happy feet over his hikes and lives for his meals and couch cuddles. Two weeks ago, the vet checked in with us to see what happened with him as she hadn't heard from us. She was so baffled when I told her he is happy and healthy and going for hikes that she insisted he come in for a free check-up because she was genuinely curious as to how he was still alive.

We took him in and she ran blood tests and checked his heart and found that the pancreatitis and fluid build up had both gone. Befuddled, she sent him home with a clean bill of health. I don't know if it was the CBD oil, my homemade diet, or Astro's sheer will to not leave me to deal with the new presidency alone, but he will be taking his CBD every day until he's no longer with me. And it's a double benefit because when I have a panic attack, we take it together!"

E.J. Duff-Berger – February 22, 2017

I have been struggling with intractable insomnia and chronic pain for nearly a decade. I have tried all manner of pharmaceuticals with little to no relief (particularly for insomnia). While I have had to take a substantial amount, this product is quite literally the only thing I have found that has provided any consistent improvement in my sleep quality and has also allowed me to begin weaning off of other drugs for chronic pain and muscle spasm. I am very thankful and excited to see how things improve over a longer period of time. Many thanks!

Zack, July 7, 2017, regarding Health 25 Imbue CBD

Research shows that CBD benefits include:

- Anti-inflammatory
- Anti-convulsant
- Anti-oxidant
- Anti-emetic
- Anxiety relief
- Anti-psychotic agent
- It can stimulate appetite
- Anti-tumor effects
- Antioxidant and neuroprotective benefits - "Cannabinoids as antioxidants and neuroprotectants" - the Abstract for the US patent (US 6630507 B1), awarded in October of 2003, reads: Cannabinoids have been found to have antioxidant properties, unrelated to NMDA receptor antagonism. This newfound property makes cannabinoids useful in the treatment and prophylaxis of a wide variety of oxidation-associated diseases, such as ischemic, age-related, inflammatory and autoimmune diseases. Cannabinoids are found to have particular application as neuroprotectants, for example in limiting neurological damage following ischemic insults, such as stroke and trauma, or in the treatment of neurodegenerative diseases, such as Alzheimer's disease, Parkinson's disease, and HIV dementia. See: https://www.google.com/patents/US6630507
- Helps to reduce the growth of aggressive human breast cancer cells and reduce breast cancer cell invasiveness:

[Cannabidiol as a novel inhibitor of Id-1 gene expression in aggressive breast cancer cells | Molecular Cancer Therapeutics](#)

CBD is a potential medicine for:

- Treatment of neuro-inflammation
- Dementia
- Epilepsy
- Glaucoma
- Pain
- Headaches
- Insomnia
- Irritable Bowel Syndrome
- Crohn's Disease
- Vomiting
- Nausea
- Anxiety
- Autism
- Schizophrenia
- Cancer
- Diabetes
- Addictions
- Alzheimer's Disease
- Osteopenia
- Osteoarthritis
- Osteoporosis
- Multiple Sclerosis
- Controlling Cholesterol

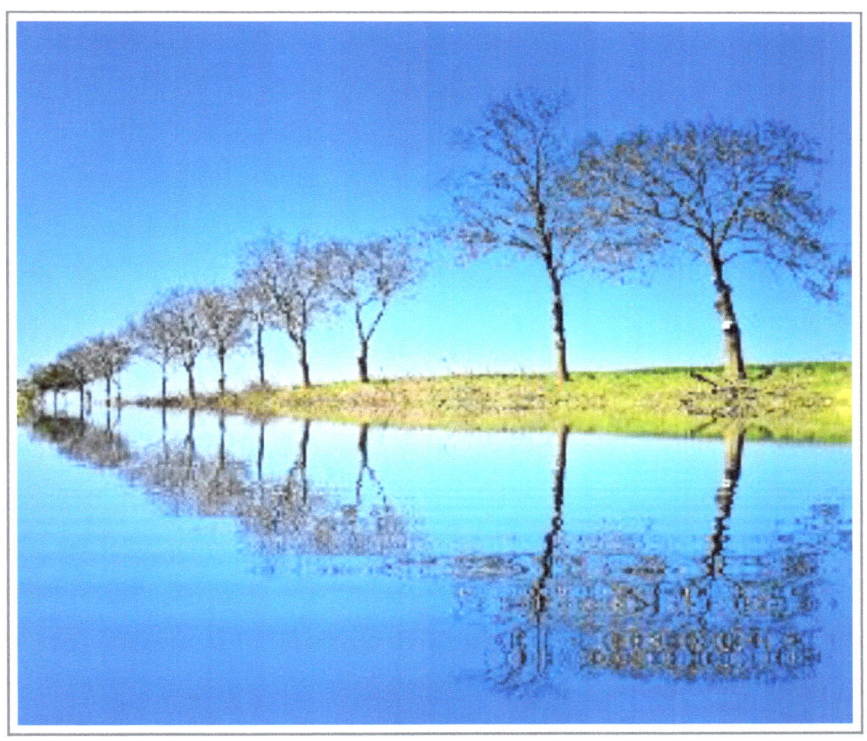

"After one week, (my Dad had) a noticeable improvement in anxiety and agitation. If only I knew about CBD earlier! If you have a loved one with Alzheimer's, I urge you to try these immediately.... It's really the only natural hope . . . and hopefully a cure to this awful disease. Thanks to the high quality CBD by Imbue Botanicals... I'll be trying the salve next!!!"

Ronda – September 20, 2016

Understandably, this new health miracle CBD is popular, and getting more so every day! Look at this excerpt from a study on colon cancer from 2013 that was published in PubMed: "CBD ... attenuates colon carcinogenesis and inhibits colorectal cancer cell proliferation..." Phytomedicine. 2014 Apr 15;21 (5): 631-9. doi: 10.1016/j.phymed.2013.11.006. Epub 2013 Dec 25.

Inhibition of colon carcinogenesis by a standardized Cannabis sativa extract with high content of cannabidiol. - PubMed - NCBI

"As an avid runner, I look to nutritional products to help recovery time from long distance runs. Since incorporating the Imbue Botanical's "Elevated" tincture, I've noticed I recover faster after long/intense runs and workouts. Highly recommended for athletes!"

Lauren – October 15, 2016

CHAPTER 4

The Financial Side of Cannabis

Because of the momentum of positive findings from the medical community and the testimonials from people and animal success stories, there is a growing need to fill the demand for CBD in many forms (tinctures, capsules, edibles, vaporizing, transdermal patches, lotions, salves, etc.) Check out this quote from Arcview Market Research, the industry leader in cannabis market research:

"Cannabis is arguably the fastest growing industry in the world. Regulated marijuana sales in North America totaled $6.9 billion in 2016, a 30 percent increase from 2015. Sales are projected to increase to $21.6 billion by the year 2021 representing a 26 percent compound annual growth rate."
Arcview Market Research

So this explains why so many companies offering CBD products have sprung up! Unfortunately, some disreputable people are just joining the industry for the profits, and are not concerned with the quality of their CBD products. In many cases, their hemp is coming from China - since it is shipped from there to Europe. They cut corners, don't grow organically, use additives, and process the plant in ways that reduce the valuable compounds that are essential.

I have had people tell me that they tried certain brands of CBD and didn't feel anything. I've also had some tell me that they have had some kind of "bad reaction" from a certain CBD product. That is one of the main reasons I wrote this book. I know that they did not take a premium quality CBD tincture or capsule if they had those results!

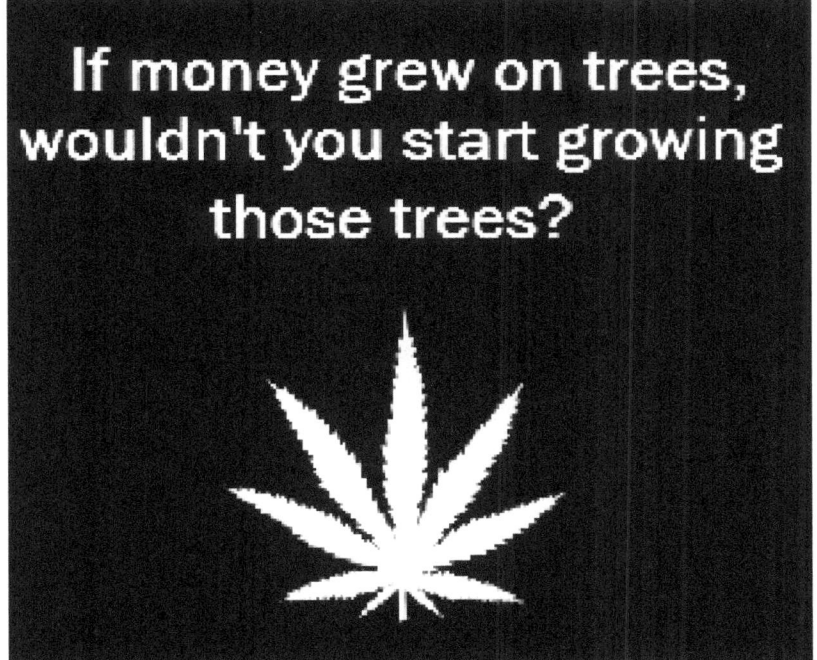

CHAPTER FIVE

What You Should Know About Your CBD Products

There are basic questions to ask any company producing CBD oil & other products such as salves, lotions, & capsules:

- Is the hemp grown in the US?
- Is your product from organically-grown hemp?
- Are they testing the soil before planting the hemp?
- Are you monitoring your plants from seed to shelf?
- What is the carrier for your tincture? Is it organic too?
- What method of processing are you using?
- How long have you been in the cannabis industry?
- Why are you in the cannabis industry?

Why is it important where the industrial hemp is being grown?
Good question!!

Answer:

When you grow hemp in the United States, you are creating a much smaller carbon footprint. It is also possible to follow the plant from the the day the seeds go in the ground and throughout the entire lifespan and harvest. *If the company has a conscience, they are testing the soil before the seeds are planted*, and doing everything according to food grade standards and making a 100% organic CBD product.

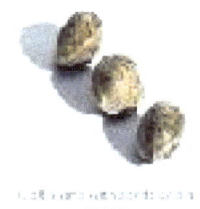 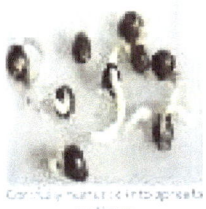 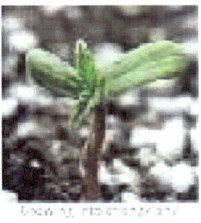 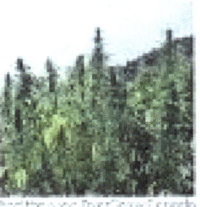

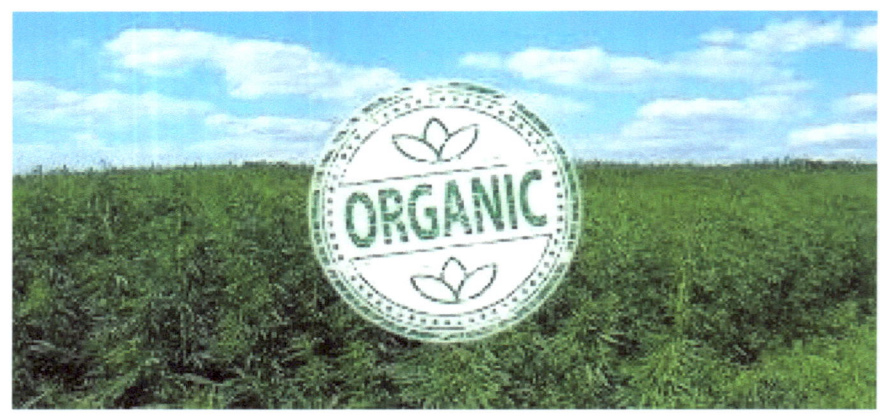

Why does it matter if the hemp is being grown organically?

Another good question!!

Answer:

Hemp is phenomenal as a phyto-remediator. It is a plant with amazing abilities to decontaminate soil. It has been used to reduce the soil toxicity around the nuclear power plant in Pripyat, Ukraine, the site of the Chernobyl disaster. The Japanese are also thinking of using hemp plants to pull the toxic metals out of the soil that was contaminated in the Fukushima meltdown.

Unfortunately, when the US occupied Japan, in 1948 they passed a Cannabis Control Law - restricting hemp from being grown. To this day it is still illegal for anyone without a license to grow hemp there, and extremely difficult to get a license! That law needs to be removed from the books so the Japanese can heal their soil and their bodies.

The following quote about Chinese-grown hemp makes one wonder how much oversight is applied to where the final hemp product ends up! Is the cadmium-contaminated hemp really going to be used for biofuel? Or is the CBD being extracted from the hemp and then shipped to Europe?

"According to a study into Chinese hemp strains conducted in 2011, many hemp strains have the ability to absorb and accumulate even large quantities of cadmium in soil without detriment to the plant itself. While *this does throw up various implications for selection of sites for cultivation of food-safe hemp*, it also indicates that cadmium-contaminated sites will particularly benefit from phyto-remediation schemes that make primary or exclusive use of hemp. Furthermore, even *if hemp used to decontaminate soil is unsafe for consumption, it can still be used in a number of industrial applications, such as for biofuel.*"

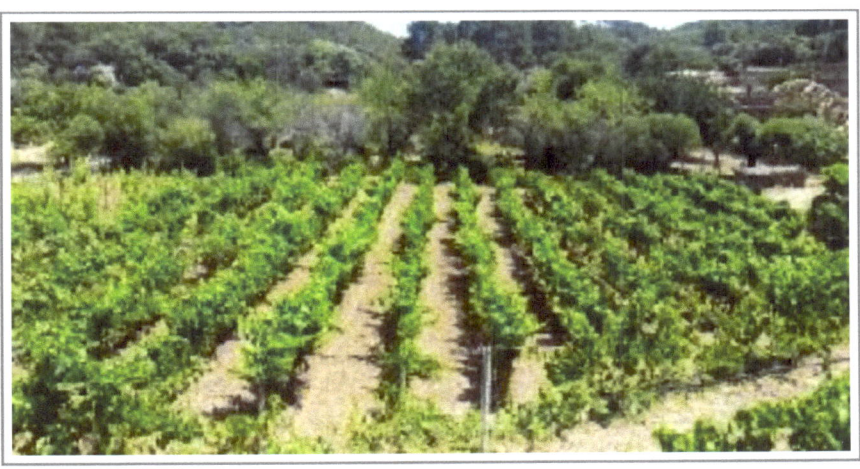

Hemp and the decontamination of radioactive soil; Sensi Seeds; Seshata, on 12/25/2013   <u>Hemp and the Decontamination of Radioactive Soil</u>

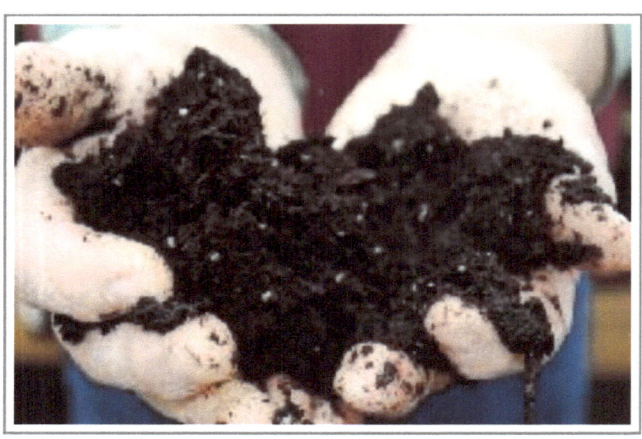

From the same story about hemp grown in China, we find the facts about cadmium contamination in foodstuffs. High levels of cadmium "can lead to joint and bone deformities, respiratory illness, anaemia, and kidney failure."

Why does it matter if the hemp harvester is monitoring their plants from seed to shelf?
That is a very good question!
Answer:
Without caring individuals tending to the soil and the planting, throughout the life of the plants and their harvest, you cannot guarantee the purity of the finished product. That's just common sense. Many companies making a variety of CBD products in the US say that the hemp they are using is "from Europe". Either they don't

really know the truth, or they are misrepresenting it. Unfortunately, in China, the CBD isolate has been extracted from the whole hemp plant and then made into a powder that is *just* CBD (cannabidiol) and none of the other beneficial cannabinoids from the plant are saved.

Then the isolate CBD powder is shipped to European countries. It is sold to companies who may be creating less than optimal quality CBD products. They may be unaware that the CBD isolate powder they are using is not organic, and for that matter it may even have toxins that are very harmful to ingest. There is concern in many segments about the quality of products coming in from China, and certainly CBD is no exception.

We already learned how suspect any CBD products from China are, and even if it were pure as the driven snow, why ship it clear across the globe? We need to grow more hemp in the US as soon as possible, and reduce the carbon footprint. Growing hemp here also has the potential to boost the economy in America and provide valuable jobs and industry.

This quote is from an article in *The Guardian*, which explains the frustration the Nebraskan farmers are feeling at being thwarted from growing hemp in their state.

"There is such a misunderstanding of hemp, it just dumbfounds me," explains Jon Hanson, an organic farmer in Marquette, who says he'd love to grow hemp on his 480-acre farm.

Unlike neighboring Colorado, where it's legal to grow such commercial marijuana strains as Purple Haze and

Chemdawg, farmers in Nebraska and elsewhere are forbidden by law from planting industrial hemp for prosaic purposes such as fiber and seed oil.

The DEA considers hemp a Schedule I drug – the same as heroin and LSD. The US Farm Bill signed by Barack Obama in 2014 carved out an exception for research and pilot programs, if states pass laws permitting it. Twenty-nine states have done so, according to the Hemp Industries Association.

But in Nebraska, a state bill to allow farmers to apply for this exception was thwarted by senators and police officials who feared hemp would be a gateway crop to recreational marijuana. An amended bill passed that limits hemp to university research.

"Anything to get the ball rolling," says former Nebraska senator Norm Wallman, a 78-year-old, fourth-generation farmer who sponsored the legislation. "You can plant it early in the spring, and it's tough as the dickens."

Dweikat says Nebraska has ideal conditions for growing hemp, which requires few pesticides and no herbicides. Driving around the state during a severe drought in 2012, he says the only green patches in the parched countryside were wild hemp plants.

John Lupien, who runs a company that separates hemp fiber from the rest of the plant, has been importing his hemp from Canada but would rather get his hemp from local farmers.

"We're stuck in the mud," Lupien says. "There are lots and lots of farmers interested in growing an alternative crop in the rotation. It would break the disease and pest cycles and have huge benefits economically and environmentally."

See the full article:
https://www.theguardian.com/us-news/2016/jun/12/
hemp-nebraska-farmers-government-block-growing-crop

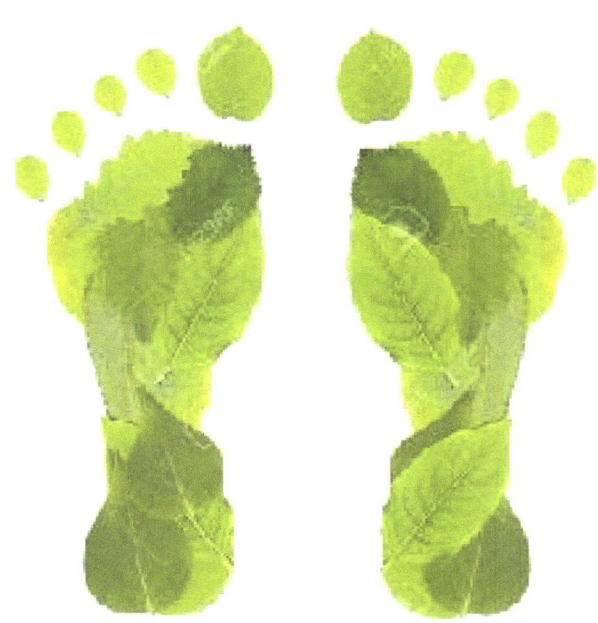

CHAPTER SIX

You Need To Know!

It is possible to get CBD analysis and contamination testing done by clean food experts. There is no excuse for any producer of premium CBD not to have it lab-tested and recorded in batches. Look for labeling which clearly shows the quantity of CBD and THC (if any) per dose, and a manufacturer's date and batch number for quality control.

CBD products should be:
- Organic - including anything in the mixture
- Verified free of mold, bacteria, pesticides
- Free of solvent residues or other contaminants
- Free of corn syrup, GMOs, trans fats, or artificial additives
- Not be undergoing extraction with solvents like BHO (Butane Honey Oil), propane, hexane, and others

Companies producing CBD products *should be happy* to answer any questions pertaining to their method of processing of the hemp. The "companies with a conscience" are doing the safest and definitely not the cheapest methods! A reputable company like Imbue Botanicals even seeks a high altitude for growing their premium hemp, to maximize the sun their plants are getting.

People "in the know" are aware of what to look for in a CBD company and they are confident with Imbue Botanicals and their attention to detail. Recently a large pharmacy group started carrying Imbue's product line. This is an excerpt from their press release:

"We are excited about introducing Imbue Botanicals to our member pharmacies, as well as entering this fast-growing market segment. We are confident that the addition of this product line for our independent neighborhood pharmacies will not only help drive revenue, but most important, will provide a whole host of alternative health solutions for our pharmacy customers.

We definitely wanted a product line that was US grown and manufactured, with a design and branding that lent itself to retail display. But we also wanted to provide a product line that provided our pharmacy customers the finest hemp CBD products on the market. We believe we found that in Imbue Botanicals."

John Pozar, Senior Vice President of Omega Legacy Group.

CHAPTER SEVEN

Care and Devotion for the Plants and the People

"We utilize a proprietary process with pharmaceutical-grade ethanol made from organic sugar cane, at low temperature and low pressure to preserve the natural cannabinoids and terpenes."

"Not all hemp is created equally. At Imbue Botanicals we utilize only our organically-grown Colorado hemp, specifically grown to be high in CBD and extremely low in THC. We grow in fields used for human-consumable crops, and most important, we grow at high altitudes (7600 feet to be precise) to maximize sun exposure, which can increase the amount of cannabinoids. Finally, we process our hemp using low temperature and low pressure to preserve the natural plant qualities."

Imbue Botanicals

Whole-plant organic hemp extract oils contain all the beneficial cannabinoids, which contain naturally occurring antioxidants and neuroprotectants. This is called 'full spectrum' in the industry. Quality processing does not heat the plant material, which would affect the final product negatively.

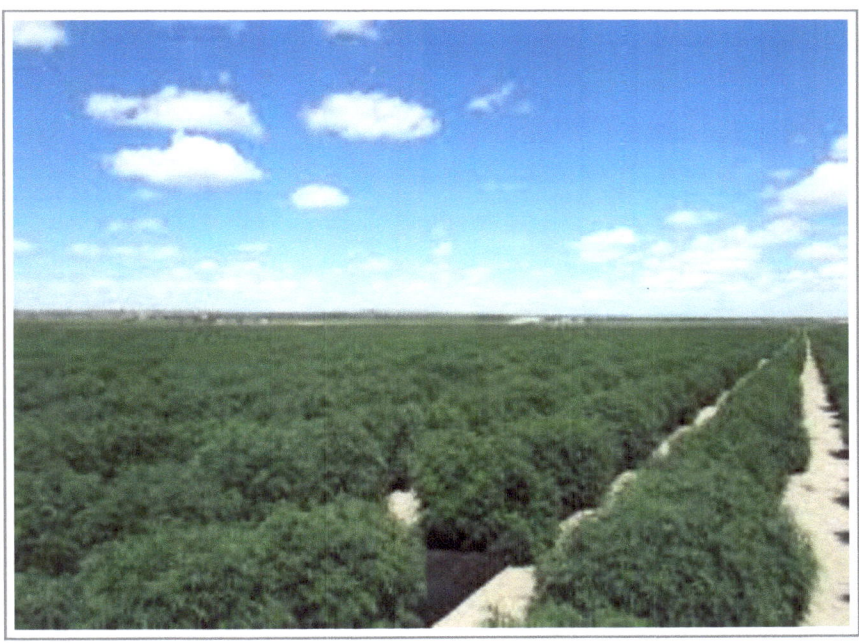

I am extremely impressed with the medicinal properties of the CBD being grown and processed by Imbue Botanicals. It can promote healing and homeostasis even in the most difficult of circumstances. It is typical for me to hear that someone did not have a good reaction to some brand of CBD, and then when I teach them about the premium CBD that Imbue

Botanicals is making, and they try it, they have a great result! This recent story tells it well:

"I had an amazing thing happen this weekend. My next door neighbor stopped over late Friday afternoon. She was outside chatting with her current visitors and the woman was upset because she has epilepsy and had her medication - but forgot her CBD - which helps stop breakthroughs.

My neighbor asked me if I would give this lady a couple of my Health-25 CBD oil capsules. I said 'sure' and bagged up 3-4 capsules, put the name "Imbue" on the bag with the dosage, and handed it off to the neighbor to give to the young woman."

Fast forward 24 hours:

"My husband come in to tell me that this couple is in the driveway and would like to talk to me! They come in and the young woman starts telling me how incredibly impressed she is by this product, which is in a league of its' own compared with anything else she has tried! Not only is it preventing a breakthrough of seizures, it also seems to make her feel carefree! She says she has never experienced anything like this! I gave them a few more capsules - she was so grateful!"

Maria Hunt ~ February, 2017
Retired Chemist for Biochemical Diagnostics, Inc.

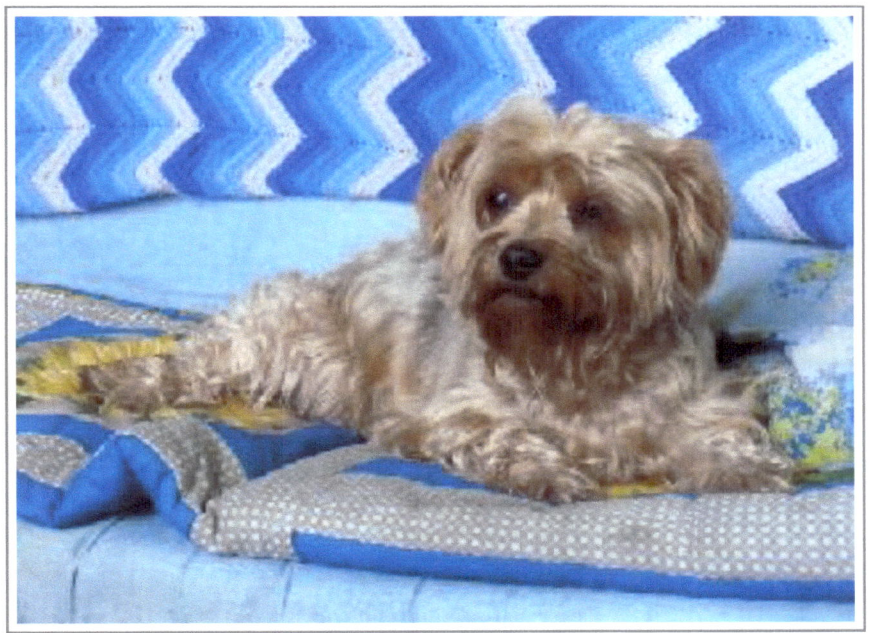

"We are a rescue, advocacy and humane education organization located in the Northeast United States. We are very impressed with quality of the product (Imbue Botanicals produces). It's an organically grown, vegan, and kosher product that is grown, sourced and manufactured in Colorado, United States.

In choosing this product line and company our demands for a product specifically for canines and felines were very high. Many companies get their source from overseas and are not organically grown. We were very happy to start seeing improvement in our seniors and those diagnosed with cancer. We're very pleased with the product thus far, and hope to continue seeing more products offered from Imbue Botanicals for both people and companion animals."

North of Boston Animal Rescue and Humane Education Society ~ October 26, 2016

"Imbue CBD truly works miracles!! The vet put my boxer on barbiturates for his seizures, but the side effects were horrible and the seizures kept coming. He's now been seizure-free for the 2 weeks that he's been taking one K-9 capsule daily. I'm so grateful to have my healthy, happy boy back! Thank you so much!!"

Jess Odin ~ November 16, 2016

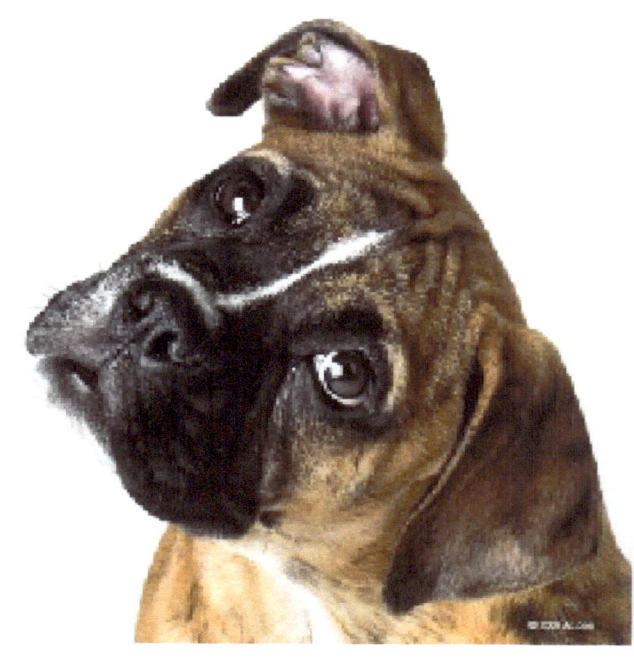

CHAPTER EIGHT

Why Does It Matter Which Carrier You Mix It With?

What difference does it make which carrier is used for your CBD tincture and is it organic too?
Answer:

This question is very important and has many facets. Some companies use flavorings and sugars in their tinctures, which is alright, if a bit sweet. And some add all kinds of unnecessary ingredients, even adding water!

Dan Iannotte, of Imbue Botanicals, wanted the tincture to be very effective and also to taste good. He insisted that it be 100% organic, not be too sweet, and be safe. The company decided to use sustainable and free trade Palm Fruit Oil for the vegetable glycerin in the tincture. Become a label reader and you will learn fast!

This is from the Imbue Botanical's tincture label-
Ingredients: Organically grown CBD Oil derived from Colorado-grown hemp and organic vegetable glycerin.

This is from a CBD tincture label from a company that is selling through multi-level marketing:

Ingredients: Sustainably & naturally grown hemp. Water, Glycerin, Phospholipids from sunflower seed oil, Ethanol, Vitamin E (as Tocofersolan and natural mixed tocopherols), Natural Citrus Oils.

Do you see the obvious differences? First off, the second one is not organic - so most likely, not safe. Second, look at all the additives that are not necessary! And water added! And this is a very high-cost product.

Dan Iannotte was asked recently **why they used Palm Fruit Oil for the glycerin, and where was it from?**

Answer:

"Malaysia."

"Why Malaysia?"

Answer:

"That's a very good question, and one that we are concerned about as well. We actually use suppliers that source their palm fruit 100% from Malaysia, utilizing only the Malaysian Pygmy Palm. Unlike Indonesia, where there are virtually no regulations on palm oil plantations and their expansion, Malaysia has a track record of creating a better approach.

In 2004, Malaysia established *The Roundtable on Sustainable Palm Oil (RSPO)*. The group, currently headed by Darrel Webber, who previously worked for the

World Wildlife Fund in Sabah, includes members from across the industry from planters to buyers, NGOs, and bankers. Together, the RSPO has created what it believes are globally credible standards covering the environment, local communities and labor standards. Those who don't comply face investigation and suspension.

So, as with all of our ingredients, we can trust this source, and use it because of the high quality standards they employ."

Thank you for your concern,
Dan Iannotte ~ Imbue Botanicals

"I recently purchased a bottle of K9 Comfort for my epileptic dog. For the past year we've been in and out of the vet trying to find a combination of meds to balance him out since he'd been seizing nearly every day since we got him.

Nothing seemed to work, in fact some pharmaceuticals actually worsened his condition. A few days ago one of the sales reps for the company (Imbue Botanicals) who is a good friend of mine suggested I try CBD oil instead; the seizures have decreased by 90% within 3 weeks and he is a much happier, healthier dog. I would definitely recommend this product and I back it 100%!"

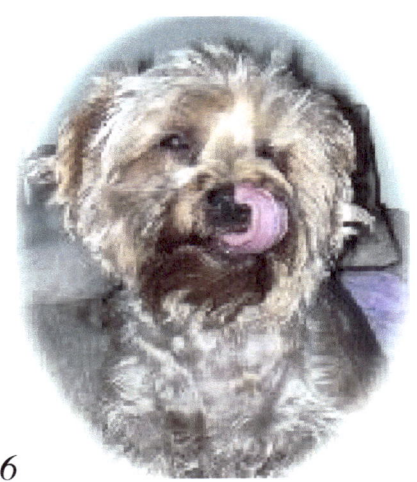

Grace ~ October 20, 2016

CHAPTER NINE

What is the Why?

And now to explore the last two critical questions: If you can talk to someone in a company who has time to answer your questions, an important one to ask is: **"How long have you been in the cannabis industry and *why* are you in it?"** Someone who is striving to cover every angle and do the best that they can do for the plant and the people has this to say:

Dan Iannotte, at Imbue Botanicals, has been researching every aspect of the cannabis industry for over 30 years. This is Dan's answer to "Why are you creating CBD products for people and pets?"

"I am in the cannabis industry because I believe the cannabis plant will not only save the world but also help make all of its inhabitants happier, healthier, kinder and more compassionate... The majority of cannabis users gravitate towards peace, love, unity, and respect."

Dan Iannotte, Imbue Botanicals

Review from Jeannette Taylor

The Imbue Botanicals Health 25mg. capsules and the tincture - and Imbue's CBD-infused Embody lotion and the Embody salve.

For the past 35 years, I've been a nurse and worked in different fields of the healing arts. I've studied complimentary medicine and gained great insight. I've concluded that the most important factor of health and healing is being OPEN MINDED.

When I was introduced to CBD oil and heard the claims and miracle stories, I had my reserve and questioned it as any scientifically trained mind would.

My story: The diagnosis and prognosis I was given in 2013 was; 2 fractured vertebrae in the lower neck with 2 herniated & degenerating discs.

I was given a life sentence by my doctors, and told I would have a life of pain and my only hope of relief would be injections every 3-6 months, and narcotic oral and topical pain management. The dosages would continue to increase as time when on. Needless to say I wasn't willing to become a slave to any addictive substance - oral, topical, OR injected!

I've suffered from the chronic neck, back, and shoulder pain for 5 years, with a constant contracted muscle tension that fluctuates by degrees as my activities vary.

Before getting in the car for a drive from Sedona to Santa Barbara, Maggie applied the Imbue Botanical's salve to my neck and shoulders. She massaged it in and within minutes the tension and pain began to subside. I instantly became a believer in the CBD MIRACLES!

I drove home and began research to see why this CBD oil works so well. To my amazement it creates homeostasis <PERFECT BALANCE> within every system of the mammalian body, seeming to go to the most out-of-balance system first. Then it makes its way to each system and helps to create balance in each one - whichever needs it the most (circulatory system, digestive system, endocrine system, lymphatic system, muscular and nervous system - you name it!)

Now for the Miracles that Imbue Botanicals products have brought to my family and friends:
* *My son's depression lifted and his energy returned.*
* *My daughter's anxiety went away; energy and creativity increased; and her eczema cleared within days!*
* *My granddaughter healed from a 2nd degree burn within 3 days.*
* *A friend with extreme sciatica who had a surgery scheduled and no feeling in his leg - he applied the*

salve before bedtime and he had feeling in his leg the next morning! He cancelled his surgery!

- *A friend with a drinking problem cut his drinking by 2/3 just by taking a Health 25 capsule 1X a day.*
- *A friend's longtime back pain subsided within minutes of applying the salve.*
- *My granddaughter's severe acne almost diminished within 3 days of applying the salve.*
- *Menstrual cramps have gone away by applying the lotion or the salve to the abdomen.*
- *My old bone and muscle injuries that have continued to linger now are gone.*
- *My headaches went away and I have a higher energy level with an overall feeling of wellness.*

This list continues to grow as I continue to share all of Imbue Botanicals' product line!

Thank you for taking the time and energy to create a truly superior CBD oil product!
Sincerely,
Jeannette Taylor
Santa Barbara Canyon Ranch

Another review about Imbue Products:
im·bue™ health25 - 25mg premium CBD capsules - 30 count
Posted By: Janelle

I have been suffering with Colitis for at least 6 years and my doctor has been treating my flare ups with several different types of anti inflammatory meds and 20 mg of prednisone, taken daily, for at least 6 weeks at a time. In the past 6 months these medicines had not been working and the pain was so intense I was having to take pain killers, which made me feel horrible everyday.

A friend of mine told me about this product, I got in touch with Maggie, who has been a Godsend in educating me on what CBD is and how it works in the body. I have also read through the website and called the guys at customer service, and they helped me figure out which product was right for me. I am a month and a half in, taking the 25mg capsules daily and have in that time, weaned myself off of the other medications entirely and feel better than ever. I have spoken to my physicians about my choice in giving CBD a try for pain relief/inflammation and they have supported this decision, even mentioning that it has been effective for many other patients. I highly recommend this product! I am finally gaining a healthy amount of weight back and feel fantastic!

In summation, I believe that for anyone who really cares about their family's health and their own, and the health of the planet, it is easy to determine which companies selling CBD products have your best interests at heart!

I feel very fortunate that I discovered Imbue Botanicals. They are doing this business with integrity and honesty. That may take longer and cost more, but it is so worth it when you see people and their pets healing! Every day I am blessed to hear another miraculous testimonial, and it is so rewarding. We are being healed and are paying it forward.

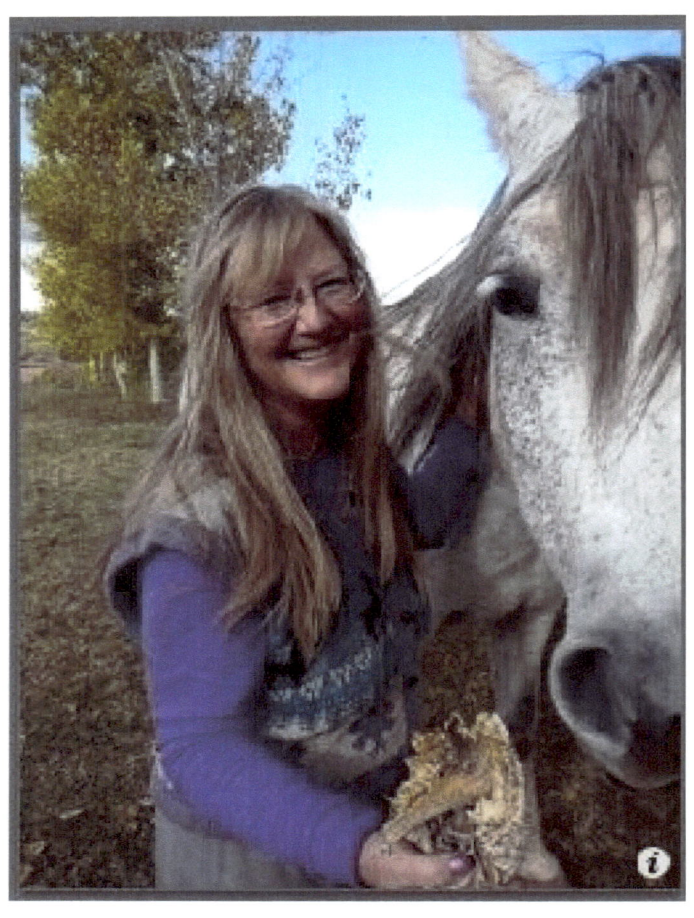

Maggie with Rein, a 13-year old pure Arabian mare, who is one of the healing horses in the small herd at Peace Tree Sanctuary.

Maggie Hall is the Founder of Peace Tree Sanctuary - A true Oasis in the High Desert - where people and animals experience a healing space to rejuvenate, recharge, and heal through the love and respect of Nature and Animals.

Peace Tree Sanctuary is a center for therapy, classes, seminars, and ceremony in Northern Arizona, in the heart of the verdant Verde Valley.

To find out more about the health benefits of CBD & Cannabis, please contact:

Maggie Hall
Peace Tree Sanctuary
maggie@imbuebotanicals.com
Phone: 844-864-6283 Ext. 720
www.imbuebotanicals.com